SONIA GONZALEZ

Vanishing Moments

The Heartbreaking Reality of Dementia

This book was professionally typeset on Reedsy.
Find out more at reedsy.com

Contents

1

Introduction

D ive into "Vanishing Moments," where we navigate the profound shifts brought on by dementia's unassuming yet life-changing presence. Embarking on "The Heartbreaking Reality of Dementia," we tread through the haze that enshrouds a silent, yet life-altering condition. Let's set the stage as we start this exploration: I'm here to shed light, not to hand out medical advice. This book is not a medical guide. Don't look here for doctor's orders or health fixes. What you're reading is a patchwork of my personal encounters, interlaced with the heartfelt struggles and insights I've gained while navigating life with dementia.

As you turn these pages, you will not find exhaustive medical research or professional healthcare directives. What you will find is a story – my story – shared with the hope that it resonates with those who are navigating similar turbulent waters. This is my narrative, woven from threads of joy and sorrow, a testament to the resilience we muster in face of life's deeply etched episodes that define our journey with this intricate ailment.

Dementia, a word that often carries a heavy burden of fear and misunderstanding, entered my life uninvited. I believe that any disease enters our lives unwanted whether it is diabetes or dementia. The intrusion of illness rewrote the script of my everyday life and transformed the core dynamics within my personal connections. I'm opening up about my journey to give you a real look at the emotional layers of living with dementia, which go way beyond what charts and clinical words can express.

This book serves as a heartfelt tribute and guide for those tending to loved ones with dementia, capturing the bittersweet essence of navigating through both challenging responsibilities and precious coherent moments.

Within these pages lies a heartfelt narrative, insights gained through trial and error, and those deeply personal instances that shape the journey of lovingly supporting someone with dementia. This book charts my journey through change, showing how embracing my own fragility led me to find strength and light in the darkest of times.

Come along on this intimate journey, where we'll look past dementia's textbook symptoms and touch the very essence of those it touches. This tale captures the essence of clinging to love even as memories slip away, shining a light on hope amid the encroaching darkness of forgetfulness and celebrating the unyielding strength of our spirit when facing dementia's daunting hurdles.

"Vanishing Moments" isn't only about what I've been through; it echoes the quiet paths so many of us tread together. In sharing my personal battles, I hope to amplify the often silent struggles we endure and bring comfort in recognizing our collective fight is never solitary. Let this book serve as your steadfast ally, offering insight and celebrating the strength we all harbor when tackling tough times.

This book is me reaching out, pulling you into my reality—a world scarred by the harsh truth of dementia but also sprinkled with deep love and surprising happiness. Let's start this adventure side by side.

2

The Beginning of the Journey

Dementia: A Simple Definition

The journey into the world of dementia often begins with a quest for understanding. Dementia isn't just one illness; it's a term that captures the steep drop in mental skills serious enough to disrupt someone's day-to-day. At its core, this illness is not a specific disease but rather a general phrase for a decline in one's mental ability that is severe enough to interfere with their daily life. Dementia often shows up as fading memory, muddled thinking, shifts in behavior, and struggles with regular tasks. While it can predominantly affect older adults, dementia is not considered a normal part of aging. Dementia springs from a whole bunch of health issues and traumas that mess with the brain. Dementia does primarily or secondarily affect the brain.

My Personal Connection

My journey with dementia began on a seemingly ordinary day. I was working from home because of Covid. It was during a casual conversation with my mom, a conversation that, unlike others, left a lingering trail of unease. The forgotten words, the misplaced memories – they were like puzzle pieces that didn't quite fit. It was the beginning

4

of a path I never anticipated walking.

Like many others, my understanding of dementia was limited to what I had seen in the media or heard in passing conversations. It was a distant concept, something that affected others but not my family, not us. That day threw me into a deep, transformative experience. It was about understanding empathy's true reach, grasping the power of love, and learning to treasure those precious moments that were quietly fading.

It feels like the person I knew and know is pulled away from you slowly. They come back for just a moment and then are pulled away again in a split second. This fluctuation between presence and absence is a heart-wrenching rhythm, a dance of connection and loss that defines living with dementia. One moment there is a spark of recognition, a familiar laugh, a shared memory, and the next, a blank stare, a confused word, a forgotten name. These moments of lucidity are both a blessing and a reminder of what is being lost.

This journey is not just about the loss of memory; it's about the loss of shared history, the gradual dissolving of the stories that have woven the fabric of our family. It's watching the person who was once the keeper of family tales and the heart of our home slip into a world where those memories no longer live. Yet, in this challenge, there is a profound lesson in unconditional love and acceptance. It's learning to love the person in front of you now, regardless of whether they remember your name or the life you've shared.

Navigating this new reality with my mom has been a journey of patience, resilience, and deep emotional learning. It has meant finding new ways to connect, creating moments of joy and comfort in the now, even as the past becomes more elusive. It's about adapting to her reality, joining her in her world, and making each interaction as meaningful as possible.

Through this experience, I've come to understand the true meaning of empathy. It's about more than understanding someone's feelings; it's about entering their world, seeing through their eyes, and feeling with their heart. It's a powerful bond that transcends memory and cognitive decline, anchored in the here and now, and in the unconditional love that underpins the relationship between a mother and her child.

The Moment of Realization

It was in the small moments that the reality of dementia began to reveal itself. The forgotten names, the repeated stories, the confusion over familiar tasks – each incident was a thread in a tapestry of change. Watching my mom struggle with these everyday occurrences was like watching a slow retreat from the world we had always known together. Although she appears to be a different person, she returns and pulls up a memory that you didn't even remember. If you ask questions about her younger days, she can tell you stories of how she and her siblings would go to dances and then to buy a soda and peanuts before they returned home. If you ask her what she had for breakfast, well, that memory is long gone. She struggles to remember what she had.

I remember the mixed emotions that came with this realization – the denial, the hope that it was just a phase, the fear of what lay ahead. We grappled with the notion that our lives were on the cusp of shifting in ways we couldn't quite wrap our heads around. The struggle is different for everyone but similar if that makes any sense.

Setting the Tone for Our Journey

This book is not a clinical exposition on dementia. Embarking on this path, you grasp the essence of sharing life and affection with a person who's traversing dementia's shifting terrain. Dementia's touch alters everything—how we adjust, how tough we stand, and the deep marks it leaves on our bonds and self-awareness.

In the chapters that follow, I will share with you not only what dementia is from a medical standpoint, but also what it feels like, what it changes, and how it reshapes the fabric of our lives. I'm about to unfold a tale that's all too familiar yet seldom shared—one of deep affection, profound grief, and the lessons these experiences teach us.

Let's take this journey hand in hand, and I'll show you how dementia is way more than a diagnosis—it's a personal saga that tugs at the heartstrings and reshapes lives from the inside out.

3

Understanding Dementia

This chapter peels back the layers of dementia, exploring its impact with clear-eyed precision. Grasping the essence of dementia is like peeling back layers from an intricate story, revealing how it quietly alters a person's reality.

Navigating the world of healthcare can often seem complex but breaking it down to its core components offers a clearer, more straight-forward understanding.

Grasping the essentials of dementia's medical side is key to truly getting the full picture of its journey. Dementia is like an umbrella. Under this umbrella are various conditions and diseases that cause changes and damage to the brain, which affects personality and language.

These ailments have a lot in common; they slowly chip away at your brainpower, mess with your memory and thinking, and make everyday stuff harder to do. While these conditions share similarities, each distinctly impacts memory and cognitive functions over time, complicating daily life. But beyond these shared symptoms, each type of dementia unfolds in its own way with distinct characteristics and timelines. Understanding this helps us appreciate why each person's experience with dementia is distinct.

Navigating the maze of dementia personally has profoundly reshaped my understanding of this complex condition.

Diving into the depths of dementia showed me its true intricacies and how it's never the same for any two people. My mom's journey started subtly – misplaced items, forgotten appointments, and occasional confusion. Initially, these seemed like simple signs of aging. However, as time passed, the changes became more pronounced. Conversations became repetitive, and familiar tasks, like using the phone, turned challenging.

Seeing her become someone I barely recognized was truly devastating. It was a gradual fading of the person I knew – a shift in her essence. As her essence slowly shifted, I learned to forge new connections, finding solace in the quiet ways we communicated and treasuring those rare moments of mutual recognition.

This transformation was not just in memory and cognitive skills, but also in the nuances of their personality. The hobbies and passions that once defined her slowly lost her allure to them. Her sense of humor, her way of expressing love, the stories she told – all began to alter, as if each day, a part of her was being erased and rewritten. Seeing her change day by day, in such profound ways, is like watching a familiar landscape shift with each passing moment—it's disorienting and deeply personal. I tell my siblings, "It is like opening a box of Cracker Jacks, you don't know what the prize is going to be for the day." Every day is different.

But within this journey of change, there were unexpected gifts. I discovered the profound depth of our non-verbal communication – a smile, a touch, a shared look – these became our new language. I found joy in the simplicity of our interactions, in the peaceful moments of just sitting together, feeling the warmth of the sun, or listening to her favorite music. These moments, though fleeting, were pockets of connection that transcended the barriers dementia had erected.

Navigating our evolving bond, I've come to see just how tough both my mom and I can be in the face of it all. Navigating through each day brought its own blend of heartache and cheer—times when grief weighed heavy, interspersed with precious flashes where mirth shone bright. Dementia's tough road led me to grasp the art of savoring every second, valuing today, and spotting splendor in these tough times. My mom is no longer the person I used to know. I am now getting to know this new person that is coming into my life.

Walking this path with my mom taught me a richer meaning of love, how to truly nurture, and the art of waiting gracefully. It showed me that even as dementia reshapes the mind, the heart can still hold onto the essence of what once was. In the face of continual loss, I learned to focus on what remained – not just the memories of the past, but the love and connection that persisted in every shared moment of our new reality.

The Emotional Impact of Early Signs

The early signs of dementia are often the hardest to come to terms with. They signal the beginning of a change, a loss that is both gradual and relentless. For me, acknowledging these signs was filled with denial and fear. I came to grips with the daunting fact that our anticipated future was veering off course. We're not just facing health challenges; we're coming to terms with our life's plot twisting in ways we never predicted.

Embracing the Journey

This chapter, and the journey it begins, is not about the clinical intricacies of dementia. We're peeling back the layers of dementia to fully understand its core, readying ourselves for the emotional journey and practical demands it entails. Keep in mind that our path ahead is not just an intellectual quest but also a deeply emotional one. We're on a path where adapting and learning go hand in hand with discovering fresh, heartfelt ways to bond.

As we move forward, we'll explore the daily shifts in living with dementia and strategies for adapting to its complex dynamics within relationships. Embarking on this path is tough, no doubt, but it's also sprinkled with genuine moments of deep connection and beauty that catch you off guard.

4

The Diagnosis

Facing the Diagnosis

The journey to a dementia diagnosis is often a road paved with uncertainty and apprehension. For many, including myself, the path begins with a suspicion, a gut feeling that something is not quite right. The road then takes us through a series of doctor visits, a mix of simple and complex evaluations, and an avalanche of inquiries—some voiced, others echoing in our heads.

A dementia diagnosis rarely comes as a single moment of revelation. Instead, it unfolds gradually, as pieces of a complex puzzle being slowly put together. The confirmation of the diagnosis is a turning point – it's a name to the unknown, a label to the experiences that have been increasingly difficult to understand.

Our Personal Story of Diagnosis

For my mom, my dad and siblings, the journey to diagnosis was a mix of emotions. There was the initial denial, the hope that it was just a phase, and the reluctance to seek medical advice. When we finally embarked on the medical consultations, it felt like stepping into a world of unknowns. The diagnosis, when it came, was a mix of relief and profound sadness. Relief, because we finally knew what we were dealing with; sadness, because of all that the diagnosis implied.

During our family's struggle, my dad becomes a pillar, gently shouldering part of the burden in looking after my mom. You see the sadness in his eyes because the person he married is no longer there. The pain in his eyes hits hard; it's clear he misses the partner he once knew. This whirlwind of change hits us all, not just me – it's tough on him and throws my siblings for a loop too.

As I opened up about the diagnosis, it became clear that its impact extended far beyond my mom—it echoed through our entire circle. Each person processed the news in their own way, but a common thread was the sense of loss – for the past and for the future we had imagined.

This shared sense of mourning brought us together in ways we didn't expect. Conversations around the dinner table shifted, becoming more reflective and supportive. We began to reminisce more, sharing stories of mom before her illness, cementing her identity in our family's narrative. These stories became a source of comfort, a reminder of the joyful moments we shared and the love that remained steadfast, despite the encroaching shadows of dementia.

The impact of the diagnosis also brought to light the strength and fragility of our family bonds. It tested us, pushed us to our emotional limits, but also revealed our capacity for compassion and empathy. We learned to lean on each other, to offer support in moments of weakness, and to find joy in the small, everyday moments that we once took for granted.

Navigating this new reality as a family was a journey of adaptation. We had to find new ways to connect with mom, to engage her in activities she could still enjoy, and to ensure that she felt loved and valued, even as her memory of us faded. We also learned the importance of self-care, recognizing that looking after our own mental and emotional well-being was crucial in being able to provide the best care for mom.

In these challenging times, our family dynamics evolved. We grew closer, our roles shifted, and we developed a new understanding of what it means to be a family facing dementia together. It was a journey marked by tears and laughter, by frustration and understanding, but above all, it was a journey of love – a love that dementia could challenge, but never diminish.

The Emotional Impact

The emotional impact of a dementia diagnosis is profound and far-reaching. It's like standing at the edge of a sea, knowing that the tide is coming in and there's no way to stop it. Standing at life's brink, you're grappling with the slow creep of loss, reshaping your tomorrows, and learning to navigate shifting roles and duties.

During this time, I really took a hard look at myself. Battling through waves of sorrow, rage, and dread, I pushed on. Yet, amidst these turbulent emotions, there was also a growing sense of resolve – a determination to face the challenges ahead with love, patience, and understanding.

Learning of my mom's diagnosis reshaped how I view her journey, and it shook the foundations of my own life as well. This realization threw me into a deep reflection on how fleeting our memories are and the transient nature of what we experience. The things that once seemed so certain - everyday conversations - were now tinged with a sense of unpredictability and impermanence.

As I watched my mom struggle with the simplest of tasks, my heart ached for the times that were no more, and for the times that were not to be. But as I faced the stark reality of her challenges, an unexpected tenacity within me came to light, steadfast and quietly powerful. It was a realization that our journey together, albeit changed, was not over. There was still so much love to give, so many moments to cherish, and new memories to create, even if they were to be remembered only by me.

Choosing to push ahead didn't erase the hurt or the anxiety, yet it laid down a solid base of optimism and bravery. It became evident that dementia could take away many things.

Embracing this new reality meant learning to find joy in the present moment, to celebrate the small victories, and to find peace in the simple, quiet moments of companionship. It was a journey of continual adaptation, not just for my mom, but for myself – redefining my role as a caregiver and learning to navigate the emotional landscape that comes with this disease.

During this time of transition, I learned the true value of reaching out and connecting with peers facing similar struggles, finding strength in our shared journey as I relied on loved ones for support. Through this shift, I've come to value the strength found in mutual support and the clarity gained from shared struggles.

Looking Ahead

As this chapter closes, we stand at the threshold of a new reality. The diagnosis of dementia is not the end; it's a new beginning. Embarking on this path with dementia is a dual quest—nurturing our loved one and simultaneously embarking on an inward odyssey of growth and change.

As we move forward, we'll dive into the everyday realities of living with dementia, how it changes relationships, and where to find the help and resilience needed. Though the journey is challenging, we're not alone; there's solace and strength in the collective wisdom of those who've tread this path before us.

5

Living with Dementia

Daily Life Altered

Living with dementia is akin to navigating a constantly shifting landscape. Navigating each day, my mom and I face a fresh set of hurdles and surprises that come with her dementia. In our journey, my mom's daily routine gradually transformed. Simple tasks that were once second nature became complex puzzles. Time became an elusive concept, and familiar faces sometimes turned into question marks. Writing a simple sentence or a name on a piece of paper became extremely difficult. The remote control for the television became the telephone. Dialing a phone number on the telephone was impossible. She told stories of people or strange animals outside that were only hallucinations. Occasionally, she's swept up by powerful waves of frustration and rage that are tough to manage. Dementia tends to turn lives upside down.

This new reality reshaped not only her world but mine as well. The way I communicated with her had to change — I learned to use simple, direct sentences and to rely more on non-verbal cues like gentle touches and reassuring smiles. Our conversations, once filled with discussions about current events or shared memories, now revolved around immediate, tangible experiences like the taste of her favorite food or the scent of fresh flowers.

Mealtimes and even her favorite foods became a challenge. Foods she once loved no longer appealed to her, and at times, she couldn't recognize what was on her plate. I had to get creative, finding new recipes and adapting meals to ensure she got the nutrition she needed. There were times when she flat out refused to eat. We all know that is not good for diabetics so corn dogs and peanut butter and jelly sandwiches became a new staple in our house. There were times that I had to turn to calling friends or family to convince her to eat while they spoke with her over the phone. Sometimes that worked and sometimes it didn't work.

Sleep patterns were another hurdle. Nights became unpredictable. Sometimes she would wander around the house, restless and confused. There were times when I would wake up to find her dressed and ready to go "home," unable to recognize that she was already there. We adapted by creating a safe, comfortable environment in the house, with night lights and easy-to-navigate spaces. We had to child proof the house so that she would not turn the stove on. We added a doorbell in case she managed to open the front door and wander out at night. She would keep us up all night sometimes for 5 days in a row. Then, things would go back to normal for a week or two if we were lucky. In my experience, she would go through spurts of being fixated on one thing for an entire week and then the next week it would be something different. What I mean by that is, if she was looking at a cow on top of the church across the street, she would want to find a way to get it down and there was no redirecting her. Everyone always told me, "You need to redirect her attention to something else when she is doing that." That never worked for her, she was stubborn and there was no way you were going to redirect her. For those of you going through what we are going through, every individual who has dementia is different. You must be creative and find what works for your person. What might work for one person might now work for another person.It is trial and error. Don't feel bad, that is just how it is.

Amidst these challenges, there were moments of unexpected joy and connection. Music became a bridge when words failed us; old songs would spark a glimmer of recognition and bring a smile to her face. Looking through old photo albums together, we could share a connection, even if she couldn't remember the names of the people in the pictures.

As her caregiver, I had to learn to be patient, to manage my expectations, and to find strength in moments of calm and connection. I also had to recognize the signs of caregiver burnout and remember to take care of myself. Finding a support network of friends, family, and professional caregivers was crucial to maintaining our quality of life.

Living with dementia is a journey of constant adaptation. It's about finding new ways to connect, embracing the present moment, and learning to ride the waves of change with grace and compassion. It's a path that requires resilience, love, and an unwavering commitment to the person behind the disease.

Navigating Daily Challenges

As a caregiver, adapting to these daily challenges requires patience, creativity, and resilience. I learned to establish a routine that accommodated my mom's changing abilities, focusing on what she could do rather than what she couldn't. We adapted by breaking down activities into simple, clear-cut steps to keep them engaging and achievable. Sometimes that was even impossible. No two days are quite the same; each brings its own set of challenges and opportunities.

Talking to my mom became tough, but I started picking up on the little things – a nod or even just a half-smile. As my mom's ability to express herself verbally diminished slowly, I learned to read non-verbal cues – a glance, a gesture, a smile. Through this journey, I've grasped the subtle art of being present — offering an ear and unwavering support without a word, amid our silent conversations. I also had to find a way to learn to deal with the frustration that I was feeling.

Maintaining Connection and Identity

Amidst the cognitive decline, it's crucial to remember that the person with dementia is still there, with their own needs, feelings, and experiences. We found joy in small moments – listening to favorite music, looking through old photo albums, or just sitting together. Engaging in these small acts, we rediscovered a comforting routine.

The Caregiver's Journey

Caregiving is a role that comes with its own set of challenges. Caring for others is rewarding, but it can also leave you feeling wiped out and on the brink of burnout if you're not careful. I learned the hard way that taking care of myself was not a luxury, but a necessity. I made it a point to carve out moments for me, reach out to my circle of friends and family, and just let the waves of feeling wash over me as they came with the job's territory. Crying seems to unleash when I finally sit down at the end of the day, watching a commercial can make me cry. I came to realize that it wasn't the commercial that was making me cry, it was the overwhelming sadness that came over me when I was thinking about my mom and dad.

Embracing the New Normal

Living with dementia means continuously adapting to a 'new normal.' It's about finding balance, seeking support, and cherishing the good days while navigating the tough ones. Navigating dementia's path challenges our endurance, yet it also uncovers the profound ways we can express care and kindness.

This journey has taught me that the 'new normal' is not static; it evolves as the condition progresses. Each phase brings its own set of challenges and demands flexibility in ways I never imagined. Simple routines become intricate exercises in patience and creativity. Finding joy in small accomplishments, like a moment of clarity or a shared laugh, becomes essential. These moments, fleeting as they may be, are what we hold onto.

Moreover, living with dementia has deepened my understanding of empathy and compassion. I've learned to see the world through my loved one's eyes, to understand their fears and frustrations, and to respond with kindness. It's a learning process to communicate effectively, to offer support without taking away their sense of independence and dignity.

Embracing this 'new normal' also means preparing for the future. It involves having difficult conversations about care preferences, legal matters, and end-of-life wishes. While these topics are challenging, addressing them early helps ensure that decisions align with my loved one's values and desires, providing peace of mind for everyone involved.

In essence, living with dementia is a journey of constant adjustment and reevaluation. It's about finding a balance between caring for a loved one and taking care of oneself. It's about navigating the tough days with resilience and cherishing the good ones with gratitude. Above all, it's a testament to the enduring power of love and the profound impact of compassion and empathy in the face of adversity.

Moving ahead, we'll explore how relationships evolve, tackle the complex healthcare maze, and confront dementia's tough later stages. Keep in mind, you've got company on this road—even when the twists and turns of dementia care seem overwhelming.

6

Changing Relationships

The Transformative Impact of Dementia on Relationships

Dementia, with its slow progression, has a profound impact on relationships. As my mom's condition evolved, so did our relationship. The roles we once held shifted dramatically. I was no longer just a child; I became a caregiver, a protector, a memory-keeper. This transformation was not immediate, nor was it easy. The road was tough, peppered with losses that cut deep, yet it unexpectedly forged stronger bonds between us.

Navigating the Emotional Landscape

One of the most challenging aspects of this journey was dealing with the sense of grief. Grieving for someone with dementia is complex because it is a loss that occurs in slow motion. You grieve for the memories they lose, for the changes in their personality, for the future you had imagined that now will be different. Grasping this kind of sorrow, the kind we call ambiguous loss, is a real journey. It asks for guts to face it and peace with what can't be changed.

Navigating through my sorrow, I found it vital to discover strategies that helped me make sense of the loss. It involved expressing my emotions, whether through writing, talking with friends or support groups, or sometimes just allowing myself to cry. It was essential to acknowledge these feelings as a natural part of the journey.

As the days turned into months and then years, this grief evolved. Grief morphed into a constant echo in my life, anchoring the bond I shared with my mom. I learned that grief is not something to be overcome or resolved, but rather something to be integrated into my life. This enduring connection, unshaken even by the fog of dementia, stood as a tribute to our shared history.

Navigating this grief also meant finding moments of gratitude amidst the sorrow. Gratitude for the times we shared before dementia, for the lucid moments that still sparkled like gems, and for the new, tender connections we formed as we walked this path together. The weight of sorrow didn't vanish, but a heartfelt thankfulness for the shared road offered comfort and perspective.

Swapping stories with others walking the same road was a game-changer. At support group meet-ups and local events, I tapped into a common dialogue about overcoming hardship and bouncing back stronger. In these gatherings, I found common ground, a place where my emotions were not only shared but also acknowledged as valid. They taught me that while each journey with dementia is unique, the emotions that accompany it are universally felt. Although I did not attend support groups often, I did find some similarities in stories told by others. I did not attend often, but I want others to know that it is important for your well-being to find support from others.

Navigating through grief, I discovered not only my own resilience but also the incredible ability of our hearts to evolve and embrace new forms of affection. This experience revealed my own resilience and the remarkable ability of our hearts to heal, evolve, and embrace new forms of affection. Loss, as tough as it is, taught me that there's always something to learn and new ways to grow in understanding each other—kind of like piecing together a giant puzzle of human emotions.

Navigating grief, we honor what was, cherish the now, and boldly shape what's to come. This path we tread is woven with not just the threads of sorrow but also those of affection, insight, and an unyielding human resilience.

Maintaining a Meaningful Connection

Despite the challenges, it's important to maintain a connection with your loved one with dementia. This connection, however, may look different than before. Being there with them, soaking up the joy in their grins and feeling soothed by their chuckles is what it's all about. Watching that smile when someone uses video call to connect with her.

Simple activities can become avenues of connection – like going for a walk, listening to music together, or engaging in simple crafts. Unlocking paths to bond and share without relying on spoken language is key. During those times, it was profoundly comforting to see that joy and serenity hadn't eluded my mom, even amid everything. But it's not a given; sometimes what we envision while reading never quite shows up on the screen. Things that used to be easy are no longer easy but mentally draining for them. Coloring can become a daunting task when they can't choose what color to use and where to use it.

Adapting to a New Kind of Love

As the disease progresses, the way we express, and experience love also changes. It shifts from exchanging words to sharing experiences that resonate without speech. It's about learning to love the person as they are now, not as they were before. This adaptation is not a subtraction of love, but rather an evolution of it.

Looking Ahead

As we close this chapter, it's important to remember that while dementia changes relationships, it does not diminish their value. Treading this road takes a heart open to change, endless patience, and deep-rooted love.

Remember, in the world of dementia, love does not forget. It adapts, growing with the constant shifts and turns life throws its way.

7

Navigating the Healthcare System

The Healthcare Maze

Navigating the healthcare system with a loved one who has dementia can feel like walking through a labyrinth. When my mom was diagnosed, I quickly realized that finding the right care and support was not a straightforward path. Navigating my mom's healthcare meant scheduling countless doctor visits, weighing various treatment paths, and choosing the best long-term care strategy. Now, I have decided to continue to care for my mom. Other options are on the backburner for now. Life is not easy when dementia is in the mix. Maybe another book will come when it comes time for long term care.

Advocating for Your Loved One

Advocacy is a crucial role for any caregiver. It means being the voice for your loved one when they can't speak for themselves. Juggling schedules with doctors and nurses, keeping tabs on meds, and having to make those hard calls is all part of the gig.

Digging into the details really paid off when it came to making smarter choices. Grasping dementia's fundamentals, weighing various therapies, and scouting care homes gave my choices a sharp edge. This also meant we had to be clear about our legal entitlements and ready to advocate for them firmly. I did find that there are not a lot of easily accessible resources when you live in rural areas. I won't discuss too much on this topic.

Finding Support and Resources

Finding support is essential for navigating this journey. In the thick of things, having people you can lean on—whether it's sharing a coffee or swapping stories over a screen—turns out to be priceless. Groups like these turned into real game-changers, dishing out not just advice but also a kind of understanding only those on the same journey could offer.

A whole host of supports await caregivers, from educational aids to break-offering services, helping them navigate their responsibilities with ease. Mastering these tools is key to navigating caregiving hurdles effectively.

Looking Ahead

As this chapter concludes, remember that navigating the healthcare system is a journey. Brace yourself for the twists and turns of healthcare; it's a path where resilience, inquisitiveness, and adaptability become your best assets.

Looking after a loved one's health means more than just securing top-notch care; it involves choosing a path that honors their self-respect and comfort, amidst the emotional whirlwind you're facing as their support system.

8

Reflections and Moving Forward

A Journey Through Heartache and Love

As we come to the close of this journey in "Vanishing Moments: The Heartbreaking Reality of Dementia," it's a time for reflection. Embarking on this path, I've weathered profound sorrow, navigated daunting challenges, and grown immensely along the way. Through the progression of my mom's dementia, we navigated uncharted waters, faced unexpected storms, and found moments of serene beauty during turbulence. Amidst the ebb and flow of her dementia, my mom's presence continues to anchor us as we strive to keep the past alive and forge new moments worth treasuring.

Navigating the journey has taught me invaluable lessons that I carry with me into every new chapter.

Navigating through dementia has granted me profound insights into life's complexities and the true essence of endurance. Navigating the twists of dementia, I've come to recognize not just how we bounce back from adversity but also the courage found in moments of openness and the deep impact of offering love without conditions. Embracing the now, finding joy in the understated moments, and acknowledging how patience and empathy can be powerful — these have become pivotal to my growth. In the midst of life's ups and downs, I've found that my faith has been a rock, offering comfort and resilience when times get tough.

Amid the chaos, I found tranquility and a renewed sense of mission through this profound bond. When things get tough, love and hope stick around, rising above the mess we face down here. Turning to prayer, meditation, or simply sitting in quiet reflection became not just a source of comfort, but also a wellspring of inner strength. It anchored me, whispering that I wasn't flying solo here and hinting at a grander scheme playing out just beyond my grasp.

Life's taught me that when we're hit with loss, we're not just stuck in place—we can actually climb to new heights from there. That during sorrow, there is space for love to flourish in new and unexpected ways. Navigating dementia's landscape, fraught with heartache and loss, surprisingly paved paths for deep emotional enrichment and soulful awakening. Navigating through dementia's challenges, I learned to appreciate the deep connections that stay intact, untouched by the erosion of memories.

Walking this journey, I've come to grasp that true love asks for nothing in return; it simply exists, unwavering and generous. It's a love that does not rely on shared memories or reciprocal expressions but is rooted in the simple act of caring, being present, and showing empathy. It's a love that endures even when the person you know seems to be fading away.

This experience really drove home how much we lean on each other and the strength that comes from our collective stories. This experience taught me that it's our shared vulnerabilities which unite us, revealing a common thread in the human condition. When we open up about our highs and lows to others who understand the caregiving journey, it builds a community grounded in compassion and collective strength.

Grasping dementia's tough teachings, I saw how it shakes our world yet underscores the indomitable strength of human resolve. This constant reminder that each day is a precious gift encourages us to embrace every chance we get to spread kindness and allows our faith, empathy, and insight to flourish amidst life's trials.

The Importance of Awareness and Support

This book was written not only as a personal narrative but also as a call to action. Dementia, this widespread ailment, still hides behind a veil of myths and social taboos. Boosting awareness, pouring more resources into research, and nurturing empathy and understanding are essential steps in the fight against dementia.

I urge you to stand up for those impacted by dementia and spread the word about its effects. Tell your tale, back up scientific studies, and foster a circle of support that gets it—there for those hit hard by dementia.

9

Conclusion

oving Forward with Hope

As we move forward from here, let us do so with hope. Let's move ahead with optimism, aiming for breakthroughs in treatments, stronger support networks, and a world that welcomes those living with dementia with open arms and hearts. Hope is not just a passive wish; it's an active engagement in seeking better outcomes, in advocating for advancements in care, and in building communities that understand and support the unique needs of those touched by dementia.

This journey does not end with the closing of this book. The ripple effects of dementia touch everyone, sparking ongoing research and inspiring both the stories we share and the steps we take to drive change. It's about more than just the scientific pursuit of a cure; it's about societal shifts towards inclusivity, empathy, and comprehensive support systems. It's about transforming our collective approach to mental health, aging, and caregiving.

As we advocate for these changes, let's also celebrate the victories, no matter how small they may seem. Each act of kindness, every moment of connection, and all efforts to raise awareness contribute to a larger tapestry of change. It's in these actions that hope finds its truest expression, fueling our continued journey towards a future where dementia no longer signifies loss, but rather challenges met with compassion, understanding, and a community ready to support.

Let this book serve as a beacon, illuminating the paths of those who navigate the murky waters of dementia. May it inspire conversations, foster understanding, and ignite a collective movement towards a world where every individual, regardless of their cognitive state, is valued, respected, and given the opportunity to live with dignity.

Together, let's embrace this cause with open hearts, armed with the knowledge that our efforts today lay the groundwork for a brighter, more inclusive tomorrow. The journey continues, and with each step we take, we carry the light of hope, guiding the way for ourselves, our loved ones, and the generations that follow.

A Parting Message

To those who walk this path, know that you are not alone. Although your journey's peppered with hurdles, it's equally rich in close relationships and meaningful experiences. Carry forward the lessons learned, the love shared, and the resilience built. And remember, in the world of dementia, every moment – no matter how fleeting – is precious.

"Vanishing Moments" is not just a title; it's a reminder to cherish every moment, to find beauty in the now, and to continue moving forward with love, understanding, and hope.

If you find that this book has been helpful to you, I'd be very appreciative if you left a favorable review on Amazon.

References

OpenAI. (2024). ChatGPT conversation on January 25, 2024. Retrieved from https://openai.com/chatgpt

Content at Scale, Inc. (2024). *Content at Scale* [Content generation service]. Retrieved from https://www.contentatscale.ai